From Gut to Glory

Nourishing Your Way to Optimal Brain Function

By Dr. Meda Ben

Table of contents

Introduction

Welcome to "From Gut to Glory: The Role of Nutrition in Brain Function," where we embark on a journey into the fascinating world of the Gut-Brain Connection—a profound link that intertwines our digestive system with the intricate workings of our brain. In this introductory chapter, we'll provide an overview of what lies ahead, the profound significance of nutrition in wellness, and a glimpse of the enlightening topics we'll explore throughout this ebook.

Welcome and Overview of the Gut-Brain Connection

The Gut-Brain Connection, often referred to as the Gut-Brain Axis, is a dynamic and intricate communication network that bridges the gap between our gut and our brain. It's a relationship that influences not only our physical health but also our emotions, mood, and cognitive function. In the chapters that follow, we'll unravel the mysteries of this connection, diving deep into its mechanisms and understanding its profound implications for our overall well-being.

The Significance of Nutrition in Wellness

At the heart of our exploration lies the central role of nutrition. What we eat has a direct and powerful impact on the harmony of the Gut-Brain Axis. The foods we choose to nourish our bodies can either promote a flourishing connection or disrupt its delicate balance. Understanding the pivotal role of nutrition in this relationship is the key to unlocking the path to optimal health and vitality.

A Preview of What's to Come

As you journey through the pages of this ebook, you'll discover a wealth of insights and practical guidance. We'll delve into the anatomy and physiology of the digestive system, explore the remarkable world of gut microbiota, and unravel the mysteries of brain structure and function. You'll gain knowledge on dietary choices that nurture both your gut and your brain, and we'll delve into lifestyle factors that play a pivotal role in maintaining this vital connection.

But that's not all. We'll provide you with practical tools, including sample recipes, meal plans, and valuable resources to empower you on your Gut-Brain Health journey.

So, whether you're seeking to enhance your well-being, boost your mood, or simply satisfy your curiosity about the profound relationship between your gut and your brain, I invite you to join us on this enlightening adventure. Let's embark on a voyage from gut to glory, exploring the transformative power of nutrition in unlocking the full potential of your Gut-Brain Connection.

Chapter 1

The Gut-Brain Axis Unveiled

The Gut-Brain Axis (GBA) is a multifaceted, intricate network of communication pathways between two of the most critical systems in the human body: the gastrointestinal (GI) tract and the central nervous system (CNS), which includes the brain and spinal cord. This chapter takes you on a journey through the heart of the GBA, unraveling its definition, revealing the profound interconnectedness between the gut and the brain, and tracing the significant historical milestones that have shaped our understanding of this extraordinary connection.

Defining the Gut-Brain Axis

The Gut-Brain Axis is a concept that captures the dynamic exchange of information between your gut and your brain. This axis involves various mechanisms through which these two essential systems communicate:

Nervous System: The gut and brain are directly connected via the vagus nerve, a major component of the autonomic nervous system. This nerve allows for real-time communication between the gut and the brain, influencing processes like digestion, mood, and immune responses.

Hormones: The endocrine system facilitates communication through hormones. For instance, when you eat, the gut releases hormones like ghrelin (stimulates hunger) and leptin (signals fullness), sending messages to your brain about your nutritional status.

Immune System: The immune cells in the gut can produce signaling molecules that influence both gut and brain health. Chronic inflammation in the gut, for example, has been linked to neuroinflammation and brain disorders.

Understanding the Gut-Brain Axis means grasping the idea that your gut and brain are in constant conversation, influencing each other's functions and ultimately, your overall well-being.

The Intricate Relationship Between Gut and Brain

To truly appreciate the Gut-Brain Axis, we must acknowledge that this relationship extends far beyond mere communication; it's a partnership that profoundly affects various aspects of our lives:

The Enteric Nervous System (ENS): The gut contains a vast network of neurons and neurotransmitters known as the ENS. Sometimes called the "second brain," this neural network can control many digestive functions independently of the central nervous system. However, it also interacts with the brain via the GBA.

Emotional Well-Being: The gut-brain connection influences mood and emotions. For instance, serotonin, a neurotransmitter primarily associated with mood regulation, is largely produced in the gut. Changes in gut health can impact serotonin levels, affecting mood and mental health.

Physical Health: The GBA plays a vital role in regulating appetite, digestion, and nutrient absorption. A healthy gut can lead to improved nutrient absorption, which can enhance brain function and overall vitality.

Historical Milestones in Gut-Brain Research

The journey of understanding the Gut-Brain Axis is a testament to human curiosity and scientific exploration. It's marked by significant milestones that have transformed our comprehension of this complex connection:

Ancient Observations: Early civilizations recognized the importance of digestive health. Ancient Greek and Roman scholars noted that gut-related issues often coincided with changes in mental well-being, highlighting the connection between the gut and the brain.

Enteric Nervous System Discovery: In the 19th century, scientists began to identify the ENS, revealing that the gut possesses its own neural network. This discovery laid the groundwork for understanding the gut's autonomous control over digestion.

Neurotransmitters and Gut: The 20th century saw groundbreaking research into neurotransmitters like serotonin and their influence on both mood and digestion. Scientists started to unravel how these molecules were essential in regulating gut-brain interactions.

Gut Microbiota Research: In recent years, the focus has shifted to the gut microbiota—the diverse community of microorganisms living in the gut. Research has unveiled the profound impact of these microbes on gut-brain communication, mental health, and overall well-being.

As we continue this exploration of the Gut-Brain Axis, the chapters ahead will build upon these historical insights. We'll delve deeper into the latest discoveries and practical applications of this connection, empowering you with the knowledge and tools to optimize the health of both your gut and brain.

Chapter 2

The Gut: Your Body's Epicenter

In this chapter, we'll embark on a detailed exploration of the gut, often referred to as the body's epicenter of health. We'll journey through the intricate anatomy and physiology of the digestive system, peer into the microscopic world of gut microbiota, and uncover the remarkable processes through which the gut digests and absorbs nutrients.

Anatomy and Physiology of the Digestive System

To understand the gut's pivotal role in overall health, it's crucial to grasp the complexity and precision of the digestive system. The digestive system encompasses a series of organs and structures that work seamlessly to break down food, extract essential nutrients, and eliminate waste. Here are some key aspects:

Mouth and Salivary Glands: Digestion begins in the mouth, where enzymes in saliva start breaking down carbohydrates. Chewing also plays a role in mechanical digestion.

Esophagus: The esophagus is a muscular tube that transports chewed food from the mouth to the stomach through a process called peristalsis.

Stomach: The stomach is a highly acidic environment where further digestion takes place. It breaks down proteins and sterilizes incoming food.

Small Intestine: This is where the majority of nutrient absorption occurs. The lining of the small intestine is equipped with tiny finger-like projections called villi and microvilli, which vastly increase the surface area for absorption.

Liver and Pancreas: These organs secrete bile and digestive enzymes, respectively, which aid in digestion and nutrient absorption.

Large Intestine: This part of the digestive system primarily absorbs water and electrolytes, while also hosting a community of beneficial gut bacteria.

A deep understanding of the digestive system's structure and function is crucial for appreciating how it contributes to the Gut-Brain Axis and overall health.

Microbiota: The Gut's Microscopic World

Within the gut lies an entire ecosystem of microorganisms, collectively referred to as the gut microbiota. This microscopic world is teeming with trillions of bacteria, viruses, fungi, and other microorganisms.

Understanding the gut microbiota is pivotal for comprehending its role in digestion and overall well-being:

Diversity and Balance: A healthy gut microbiota is diverse, with various species coexisting in a state of balance. An imbalance, often referred to as dysbiosis, can lead to digestive issues and impact overall health.

Digestive Assistance: Some gut bacteria assist in the breakdown of complex carbohydrates and fiber that human enzymes cannot fully digest. They produce short-chain fatty acids (SCFAs) that are vital for gut health.

Immune System Regulation: Gut microbiota plays a crucial role in training and modulating the immune system. A balanced microbiota can help protect against infections and autoimmune disorders.

Neurotransmitter Production: Certain gut bacteria are capable of producing neurotransmitters like serotonin and dopamine, which influence mood and cognitive function.

How the Gut Digests and Absorbs Nutrients

The digestive and absorptive processes within the gut are marvels of precision and efficiency. Nutrients from the food we consume must undergo a series of transformations to become usable by the body:

Digestion: Food is broken down into smaller molecules through mechanical and chemical processes. Enzymes and stomach acid play pivotal roles in this phase.

Absorption: Nutrients, in their smaller forms, are absorbed through the walls of the small intestine. Different nutrients, such as carbohydrates, proteins, fats, vitamins, and minerals, are absorbed in specific areas of the small intestine.

Transportation: Nutrients are transported via the bloodstream to cells throughout the body, where they are utilized for energy, growth, repair, and overall well-being.

Waste Elimination: Undigested food particles and waste products are eliminated from the body through the large intestine.

Understanding these processes is essential not only for comprehending the gut's role in nourishing the body but also for recognizing how these processes can impact the Gut-Brain Axis. In the chapters that follow, we will explore in-depth how the gut's functioning affects brain health and, conversely, how the brain influences digestive processes and overall well-being.

Chapter 3

The Brain: The Command Center

In this chapter, we'll delve into the magnificent realm of the brain, often referred to as the body's command center. Our journey will begin with an exploration of the brain's structure and function, followed by a deep dive into how brain health influences cognitive performance. Finally, we'll uncover the brain's specific nutritional needs, which play a critical role in maintaining optimal function and overall well-being.

Understanding Brain Structure and Function

The human brain is a marvel of evolution, a complex organ comprising billions of neurons interconnected in intricate networks. Understanding its structure and function is fundamental to appreciating its role in our lives:

Structure: The brain consists of several regions, each with distinct functions. The cerebrum, divided into lobes like the frontal, parietal, temporal, and occipital lobes, plays a central role in higher cognitive functions. The cerebellum controls coordination and balance, while the brainstem regulates basic life functions such as breathing and heart rate.

Function: The brain is responsible for an astonishing array of tasks, including processing sensory information, regulating emotions, controlling voluntary movements, and managing memory and learning. It is also where thoughts, consciousness, and self-awareness originate.

Neurotransmitters: Communication within the brain occurs through neurotransmitters—chemical messengers that relay signals between neurons. Key neurotransmitters like dopamine, serotonin, and acetylcholine influence mood, memory, and cognition.

Brain Health and Cognitive Performance

A healthy brain is vital for maintaining cognitive performance and overall well-being. Brain health encompasses several aspects:

Neuroplasticity: The brain's remarkable ability to adapt and rewire itself in response to learning and experience is known as neuroplasticity. This phenomenon underlies our capacity to learn new skills and recover from injuries.

Cognitive Performance: Cognitive performance encompasses various mental functions, including memory, attention, problem-solving, and decision-making. A healthy brain is essential for optimal cognitive performance.

Mental Health: Brain health is closely intertwined with mental health. Conditions like depression, anxiety, and neurodegenerative diseases can significantly impact cognitive function and overall quality of life.

Lifestyle Factors: Lifestyle choices, including diet, physical activity, sleep, and stress management, profoundly affect brain health and cognitive performance.

The Brain's Nutritional Needs

The brain is a metabolically active organ with high energy and nutrient requirements. Proper nutrition is essential to support its functioning:

Macronutrients: Carbohydrates provide glucose, the brain's primary energy source. Healthy fats, particularly omega-3 fatty acids, are crucial for brain structure and function. Proteins supply amino acids required for neurotransmitter production.

Micronutrients: A wide range of vitamins and minerals, including B vitamins, vitamin D, magnesium, and antioxidants like vitamin C and E, play vital roles in brain health.

Hydration: Adequate hydration is critical for maintaining optimal cognitive function. Dehydration can lead to poor concentration, memory problems, and cognitive fatigue.

Antioxidants: Antioxidants protect brain cells from oxidative stress and inflammation, which can contribute to cognitive decline and neurodegenerative diseases.

Phytonutrients: Plant-based compounds found in fruits, vegetables, and herbs have been linked to improved cognitive function and brain health.

As we delve further into the chapters ahead, we will explore how the Gut-Brain Axis intimately connects with the brain's well-being. Proper nutrition and the relationship between the gut and the brain are integral components of this connection, ultimately influencing mood, cognition, and overall health.

Chapter 4

Nutrients for Nurturing the Gut

In this chapter, we'll embark on a journey to understand the pivotal role of nutrition in nurturing a healthy gut. We'll explore how diet impacts gut health, identify essential nutrients crucial for a thriving gut, and discover a variety of foods that promote and support gut well-being.

The Role of Diet in Gut Health

Your dietary choices have a profound impact on the health of your gut. The foods you consume can either nurture and support a flourishing gut microbiome or disrupt its delicate balance. Here's how diet plays a crucial role in gut health:

Fiber-Rich Foods: A diet rich in dietary fiber, found in fruits, vegetables, whole grains, and legumes, provides the necessary fuel for beneficial gut bacteria. These bacteria ferment dietary fiber, producing short-chain fatty acids (SCFAs) like butyrate, which help maintain a healthy gut lining.

Prebiotics: Prebiotics are a type of fiber that selectively nourishes beneficial gut bacteria. Foods like garlic, onions, leeks, and asparagus are excellent sources of prebiotics.

Probiotics: Probiotics are live beneficial bacteria that can be found in fermented foods like yogurt, kefir, sauerkraut, kimchi, and miso. Consuming probiotics can help replenish and diversify your gut microbiome.

Sugar and Processed Foods: High-sugar and processed foods can disrupt the balance of gut bacteria, leading to the proliferation of harmful species. Reducing the intake of these foods is essential for gut health.

Artificial Sweeteners: Some artificial sweeteners, despite being low in calories, may negatively affect the gut microbiota. Research suggests they can alter the composition of gut bacteria and may not be the best choice for gut health.

Alcohol and Caffeine: Excessive alcohol consumption can harm the gut lining and disrupt the gut microbiota. Similarly, excessive caffeine intake may lead to digestive issues for some individuals.

Essential Nutrients for a Healthy Gut

Nourishing your gut goes beyond just avoiding harmful foods. Ensuring you receive essential nutrients is equally crucial for gut health:

Fiber: Dietary fiber, particularly soluble fiber, is essential for regular bowel movements, maintaining a healthy gut lining, and supporting beneficial bacteria.

Polyphenols: These plant compounds, found in foods like berries, dark chocolate, and green tea, have antioxidant and anti-inflammatory properties that can benefit gut health.

Omega-3 Fatty Acids: These healthy fats, found in fatty fish, flaxseeds, and walnuts, have anti-inflammatory effects that can help reduce gut inflammation.

Vitamins and Minerals: Nutrients like vitamin D, magnesium, and zinc play various roles in gut health, including supporting the gut lining and immune function.

Collagen: Collagen, found in bone broth and supplements, can support the gut lining's integrity and promote overall gut health.

Foods That Promote Gut Well-Being

A well-rounded diet that includes a variety of nutrient-rich foods can help promote gut well-being:

Yogurt: Plain yogurt with live cultures is a good source of probiotics that can support a healthy gut microbiome.

Fermented Foods: Foods like kimchi, sauerkraut, kefir, and miso contain beneficial probiotics that aid in maintaining a diverse gut microbiota.

Fruits and Vegetables: These are rich in fiber, vitamins, minerals, and antioxidants that promote gut health.

Whole Grains: Foods like oats, quinoa, and brown rice provide fiber and essential nutrients for gut well-being.

Legumes: Beans, lentils, and chickpeas are excellent sources of both fiber and protein, supporting a healthy gut.

Nuts and Seeds: Almonds, chia seeds, and flax seeds provide fiber and healthy fats that benefit gut health.

Herbs and Spices: Garlic, ginger, turmeric, and oregano have antimicrobial and anti-inflammatory properties that can support gut health.

Bone Broth: Rich in collagen and amino acids, bone broth can help maintain the gut lining's integrity.

Understanding how dietary choices influence gut health is the first step toward nurturing a thriving gut microbiome. By incorporating these nutrient-rich foods and making informed dietary decisions, you can promote and maintain a healthy gut, which, in turn, can positively impact your overall well-being and the intricate Gut-Brain Axis.

Chapter 5

The Gut-Brain Connection in Action

In this chapter, we will explore the Gut-Brain Connection in action, shedding light on how the gut profoundly influences brain health, how the gut microbiota impacts mood and cognition, and providing real-life examples and case studies that illustrate the remarkable interplay between these two essential systems.

The Gut's Influence on Brain Health

The gut plays a pivotal role in maintaining and influencing brain health in several ways:

Neurotransmitter Production: Your gut is a hub for neurotransmitter production, including serotonin, dopamine, and gamma-aminobutyric acid (GABA). These neurotransmitters are instrumental in regulating mood, emotions, and mental well-being. An imbalance in gut microbiota can disrupt neurotransmitter production, potentially leading to mood disorders such as depression and anxiety.

Inflammation and Immune Response: A balanced gut microbiota helps regulate the immune system and reduce inflammation. Chronic inflammation in the gut can lead to a state of chronic systemic inflammation, which has been linked to neuroinflammation and neurodegenerative diseases like Alzheimer's and Parkinson's.

The Gut-Brain Axis Communication: The gut and brain communicate through various pathways, including the vagus nerve, immune system signals, and the production of signaling molecules like cytokines and hormones. This constant dialogue influences a wide range of brain functions, including memory, cognition, and emotional responses.

How Gut Microbiota Impacts Mood and Cognition

The gut microbiota, consisting of trillions of microorganisms residing in your digestive tract, has a profound impact on mood and cognition:

Microbiota-Derived Metabolites: Beneficial gut bacteria ferment dietary fiber to produce short-chain fatty acids (SCFAs), including butyrate. SCFAs have been linked to improved mood and cognitive function, as they can cross the blood-brain barrier and influence brain health directly.

Neurotransmitter Production: Some gut bacteria are capable of producing neurotransmitters, such as serotonin and GABA. A well-balanced gut microbiota can help regulate neurotransmitter levels, positively affecting mood and anxiety levels.

The Gut-Brain Immune Connection: A balanced gut microbiota can regulate the immune system, preventing excessive inflammation that can impair cognitive function and mood stability.

Case Studies and Real-Life Examples

To illustrate the Gut-Brain Connection's real-world impact, let's delve into some case studies and examples:

Irritable Bowel Syndrome (IBS) and Anxiety: Many individuals with IBS experience comorbid anxiety. Research has shown that improving gut health through dietary changes and probiotics can alleviate IBS symptoms and reduce anxiety levels.

Depression and Gut Microbiota: Studies have highlighted significant differences in the gut microbiota composition of individuals with depression compared to those without. Interventions such as probiotics and dietary modifications have shown promise in alleviating depressive symptoms.

Dietary Interventions: Real-life examples often feature individuals who have transformed their gut health and, consequently, their mental well-being through dietary changes. These stories demonstrate the profound impact that simple adjustments to one's diet can have on mood and cognition.

Athletes and Gut Health: Elite athletes often prioritize gut health due to its potential impact on performance. Case studies involving athletes who have optimized their gut microbiota through dietary strategies can provide valuable insights into the relationship between gut health and cognitive function, as well as physical performance.

By examining these real-life examples and case studies, we gain a deeper appreciation of how the Gut-Brain Connection influences our daily lives, offering hope and actionable insights for individuals seeking to improve both their gut and brain health. Understanding this connection is a powerful tool for enhancing overall well-being and achieving a balanced and harmonious relationship between the gut and the brain.

Chapter 6

Lifestyle Factors

This chapter dives deep into the lifestyle factors that significantly influence both gut and brain health. We will explore the impact of exercise, the critical roles of sleep, stress management, and mindfulness, and the importance of staying well-hydrated.

Exercise and Its Impact on Gut and Brain Health

Exercise is a powerhouse for overall health, and it profoundly affects both your gut and brain:

Gut Health: Physical activity can positively influence gut microbiota diversity. Regular exercise has been associated with an increase in beneficial bacteria and a decrease in harmful ones. This balance can promote gut health, enhance digestion, and reduce the risk of gastrointestinal disorders.

Brain Health: Exercise is a natural brain booster. It increases blood flow to the brain, promoting the delivery of oxygen and nutrients critical for optimal cognitive function. Regular physical activity has also been linked to improved mood, reduced stress, and a decreased risk of neurodegenerative diseases like Alzheimer's.

Gut-Brain Axis: Exercise plays a role in strengthening the Gut-Brain Axis. The improved gut health and reduced inflammation associated with physical activity can enhance communication between your gut and brain, leading to better overall well-being.

Sleep, Stress Management, and Mindfulness

Quality sleep and effective stress management are paramount for maintaining a harmonious Gut-Brain Connection:

Sleep: A lack of sleep can disrupt the gut microbiota, leading to imbalances that may affect digestion and metabolism. Poor sleep quality can also hinder cognitive function, impair memory consolidation, and increase the risk of mood disorders. Prioritizing restorative sleep is essential for nurturing both your gut and brain.

Stress Management: Chronic stress can wreak havoc on the Gut-Brain Axis. It can lead to gastrointestinal problems, trigger inflammation, and contribute to mood disorders. Implementing stress management techniques, such as mindfulness, meditation, and relaxation exercises, can help mitigate these effects and support a healthy gut-brain relationship.

Mindfulness: Mindfulness practices involve being fully present in the moment and can positively influence the Gut-Brain Connection. Mindfulness-based stress reduction (MBSR) programs have shown promise in improving gut health by reducing inflammation and promoting a more balanced gut microbiota. These practices can also enhance mental clarity and emotional well-being.

The Importance of Hydration

Proper hydration is often overlooked but is vital for both gut and brain health:

Gut Health: Hydration supports regular bowel movements and helps prevent constipation. A well-hydrated gut ensures that food moves through the digestive system smoothly, aiding in nutrient absorption and overall gut health.

Brain Health: Dehydration can negatively impact cognitive function. Even mild dehydration can impair attention, memory, and decision-making. Maintaining proper hydration is crucial for ensuring that your brain functions optimally.

Gut-Brain Axis: Adequate hydration is essential for the smooth operation of the Gut-Brain Axis. Dehydration can lead to imbalances in gut microbiota and increased inflammation, potentially affecting mood and cognitive performance.

Incorporating regular exercise, prioritizing restful sleep, managing stress through mindfulness techniques, and ensuring proper hydration are actionable steps you can take to optimize both your gut and brain health. These lifestyle factors, when integrated into your daily routine, contribute significantly to a harmonious and thriving Gut-Brain Connection, promoting overall well-being and vitality.

Chapter 7

Gut Health for Long-Term Wellness

This chapter delves into the importance of maintaining a healthy gut for long-term well-being. We will explore preventive measures to support gut health, gain an understanding of common digestive disorders, and emphasize the role of regular check-ups in preserving a thriving Gut-Brain Connection.

Preventive Measures for a Healthy Gut

Proactively caring for your gut is a cornerstone of long-term wellness:

Balanced Diet: A diet rich in fiber, prebiotics, and a variety of nutrients supports gut health. Consuming a diverse range of fruits, vegetables, whole grains, and lean proteins nourishes your gut microbiota and promotes a harmonious balance of bacteria.

Probiotics: Consider incorporating probiotic-rich foods like yogurt, kefir, and sauerkraut into your diet. Probiotic supplements can also be beneficial, particularly during and after antibiotic treatments or to address specific gut health concerns.

Hydration: Maintaining proper hydration ensures that your digestive system functions optimally. Water is crucial for breaking down food, moving it through the digestive tract, and supporting nutrient absorption.

Fiber Intake: Aim to consume an adequate amount of dietary fiber daily. Fiber aids in regular bowel movements, prevents constipation, and provides nourishment to beneficial gut bacteria.

Stress Management: Implement stress-reduction techniques such as meditation, mindfulness, and relaxation exercises. Chronic stress can disrupt the Gut-Brain Axis and negatively impact gut health.

Regular Physical Activity: Engage in regular exercise to promote gut microbiota diversity and reduce the risk of gastrointestinal issues. Exercise also supports overall well-being, benefiting both gut and brain health.

Understanding Digestive Disorders

Being informed about common digestive disorders empowers you to recognize potential issues and seek timely intervention:

Irritable Bowel Syndrome (IBS): IBS is a common digestive disorder characterized by abdominal pain, bloating, and altered bowel habits. It can be triggered by stress, dietary factors, or a combination of both.

Inflammatory Bowel Disease (IBD): Conditions like Crohn's disease and ulcerative colitis fall under the umbrella of IBD. These chronic conditions involve inflammation of the gastrointestinal tract, leading to symptoms such as abdominal pain, diarrhea, and weight loss.

Gastroesophageal Reflux Disease (GERD): GERD occurs when stomach acid frequently flows back into the esophagus, causing heartburn and potentially damaging the esophagus lining.

Celiac Disease: This autoimmune disorder is triggered by the ingestion of gluten, a protein found in wheat, barley, and rye. Celiac disease damages the lining of the small intestine and can lead to malabsorption of nutrients.

The Role of Regular Check-Ups

Regular health check-ups are invaluable in safeguarding both your gut and brain health:

Preventive Screening: Routine check-ups allow for early detection and prevention of potential gut-related issues. Screening for conditions like colorectal cancer can lead to early intervention and better outcomes.

Management of Chronic Conditions: For individuals with preexisting digestive disorders or chronic illnesses, regular check-ups are essential for monitoring and managing their conditions. This proactive approach can help prevent complications and ensure optimal gut health.

Personalized Care: Healthcare professionals can provide personalized dietary and lifestyle recommendations tailored to your specific needs. Regular check-ups enable healthcare providers to track your progress and make necessary adjustments to your treatment plan.

Overall Well-Being: Remember that a holistic approach to health, which encompasses both gut and brain well-being, is essential for long-term wellness. Regular check-ups offer a comprehensive view of your health, helping you make informed decisions for your well-being.

By embracing preventive measures, understanding common digestive disorders, and prioritizing regular check-ups, you can lay the foundation for long-term gut health. This proactive approach not only contributes to a thriving Gut-Brain Connection but also enhances your overall quality of life, allowing you to enjoy lasting well-being and vitality.

Chapter 8

Implementing Change

In this chapter, we'll explore the practical steps to implement change in your life, focusing on setting realistic health goals, overcoming challenges in dietary changes, and the importance of tracking progress and making adjustments along the way.

Setting Realistic Health Goals

Setting clear and achievable health goals is the first step toward improving your gut and brain health:

Specific Goals: Be precise about what you want to achieve. Instead of a vague goal like "eat healthier," consider specific objectives like "consume at least five servings of vegetables daily" or "reduce sugar intake by 20%."

Measurable Goals: Ensure your goals are quantifiable, so you can track your progress. This might involve keeping a food journal, monitoring exercise frequency, or measuring specific health indicators.

Attainable Goals: Be realistic about what you can achieve within your current circumstances. Set goals that challenge you but are still within your reach. Gradual, sustainable changes are more likely to succeed.

Relevant Goals: Your goals should align with your broader health objectives and values. Understand why you want to make these changes and how they contribute to your overall well-being.

Time-Bound Goals: Establish a timeframe for achieving your goals. This helps create a sense of urgency and accountability. For example, you might aim to reach a certain milestone within three months.

Overcoming Challenges in Dietary Changes

Changing dietary habits can be challenging, but with the right strategies, you can overcome obstacles:

Gradual Transition: Rather than making drastic changes overnight, consider a gradual transition. Start by incorporating one healthy habit at a time, allowing your body and taste buds to adapt.

Mindful Eating: Pay attention to your eating habits and emotional triggers. Are you eating out of stress or boredom? Practice mindful eating by savoring each bite, eating without distractions, and listening to your body's hunger and fullness cues.

Support System: Share your goals with friends and family who can provide encouragement and accountability. Consider joining a support group or seeking guidance from a registered dietitian or nutritionist.

Positive Reinforcement: Reward yourself for achieving milestones along the way. Celebrate your successes with non-food rewards, such as a spa day, a new book, or a fitness-related gift.

Resilience: Understand that setbacks are a natural part of the journey. Instead of viewing them as failures, consider them opportunities to learn and adjust your approach.

Tracking Progress and Making Adjustments

Monitoring your progress and making necessary adjustments are key to sustaining change:

Record Keeping: Keep a detailed record of your dietary choices, exercise routines, and overall well-being. This information allows you to identify patterns, both positive and negative.

Measurement Tools: Use tools like food diaries, fitness trackers, and health apps to quantify your progress. These tools can provide valuable insights into your habits and help you stay on track.

Regular Evaluation: Periodically assess your goals and progress. Are you meeting your targets? Are there areas where you've encountered challenges? Reflect on what's working and what needs adjustment.

Flexibility: Be flexible in your approach. If you find that a particular dietary plan or exercise routine isn't sustainable or enjoyable, don't hesitate to modify it to better suit your needs and preferences.

Seek Professional Guidance: If you're facing persistent challenges or health concerns, consider consulting a healthcare professional, registered dietitian, or fitness expert for personalized guidance and support.

By setting realistic health goals, adopting strategies to overcome dietary challenges, and consistently tracking your progress while remaining adaptable, you can implement lasting change in your life. These steps are crucial for nurturing both your gut and brain health, ultimately leading to improved overall well-being and vitality

Chapter 9

Recipes and Meal Plans

This chapter is a treasure trove of delectable recipes and comprehensive meal plans designed to promote both gut and brain health. We'll explore sample recipes, weekly meal plans, shopping lists, and cooking tips to help you embark on a flavorful and nutritious journey.

Sample Recipes for Gut and Brain Health

Elevate your culinary experience with these delectable recipes, crafted to nurture your gut and brain:

Note: Each recipe is carefully designed to include ingredients that support gut health, provide essential nutrients for brain function, and offer a delightful dining experience.

Recipe 1: Gut-Boosting Breakfast Bowl

Ingredients:

1 cup Greek yogurt (probiotic-rich)

1/2 cup mixed berries (antioxidant-packed)

1 tablespoon honey (natural sweetener)

2 tablespoons chia seeds (fiber source)

1/4 cup granola (whole grains)

1 tablespoon almond butter (healthy fats)

Recipe 2: Brain-Boosting Salmon Salad

Ingredients:

4 oz grilled salmon (omega-3 fatty acids)

2 cups spinach leaves (folate and iron)

1/4 cup walnuts (brain-boosting nuts)

1/2 cup cherry tomatoes (antioxidant-rich)

1/4 cup avocado (healthy fats)

Balsamic vinaigrette dressing (olive oil-based)

Recipe 3: Gut-Brain Harmony Stir-Fry

Ingredients:

1 cup broccoli florets (fiber source)

1/2 cup bell peppers (vitamin C)

1/2 cup sliced carrots (fiber and beta-carotene)

4 oz lean chicken breast (protein)

1 cup cooked quinoa (whole grains)

2 tablespoons soy sauce (fermented goodness)

1 clove garlic (prebiotic)

1 tablespoon olive oil (healthy fats)

Weekly Meal Plans

Unlock the potential of these meal plans, carefully curated to provide a week's worth of nourishing meals for your gut and brain:

Day 1: Gut and Brain Kickstart

Breakfast: Gut-Boosting Breakfast Bowl

Lunch: Brain-Boosting Salmon Salad

Dinner: Gut-Brain Harmony Stir-Fry

Day 2: Nutrient-Rich Delights

Breakfast: Greek yogurt parfait with honey and almonds

Lunch: Spinach and walnut salad with grilled chicken

Dinner: Baked salmon with steamed broccoli and quinoa

Day 3: Plant-Powered Goodness

Breakfast: Berry and spinach smoothie

Lunch: Chickpea and vegetable stir-fry

Dinner: Lentil soup with whole-grain bread

Day 4: Vibrant and Balanced

Breakfast: Oatmeal with fresh berries

Lunch: Mixed greens salad with tuna

Dinner: Roasted vegetables with quinoa and tahini dressing

Day 5: Colorful Feast

Breakfast: Greek yogurt with mixed berries and chia seeds

Lunch: Quinoa and black bean salad

Dinner: Grilled chicken with sautéed spinach and sweet potatoes

Day 6: Mediterranean Delights

Breakfast: Mediterranean-style scrambled eggs

Lunch: Greek salad with feta cheese and olives

Dinner: Baked cod with roasted vegetables and couscous

Day 7: Sunday Simplicity

Breakfast: Avocado toast with poached eggs

Lunch: Caprese salad with balsamic glaze

Dinner: Lemon herb roasted chicken with asparagus

Shopping Lists and Cooking Tips

To simplify your journey towards better gut and brain health, here are shopping lists and essential cooking tips:

Shopping List Essentials:

Probiotic-rich foods like Greek yogurt and kefir

A variety of colorful fruits and vegetables for antioxidants

Lean sources of protein, including salmon, chicken, and eggs

Healthy fats like avocado, nuts, and olive oil

Whole grains such as quinoa and whole-grain bread

Fiber-rich foods like chia seeds, lentils, and broccoli

Brain-boosting ingredients like walnuts and berries

Cooking Tips:

Opt for grilling, roasting, steaming, or sautéing instead of deep frying to retain nutrients.

Experiment with herbs and spices to add flavor without excessive salt or sugar.

Practice portion control to ensure balanced meals.

Batch cooking and meal prep can save time and ensure healthier choices throughout the week.

Enjoy meals mindfully, savoring each bite and paying attention to hunger and fullness cues.

Embark on this culinary adventure, exploring these delectable recipes and meal plans while nourishing your gut and brain for long-term health and vitality. By incorporating these delicious and nutritious options into your daily life, you can enhance your well-being and embrace a harmonious Gut-Brain Connection.

Chapter 10

Resources and Further Reading

In this final chapter, we provide you with a valuable list of resources, books, websites, blogs, apps, and research studies to further your exploration of gut and brain health. These resources will empower you to continue your journey towards well-being, providing a wealth of information and tools to support your ongoing efforts.

Recommended Books

Brain Maker: The Power of Gut Microbes to Heal and Protect Your Brain by Dr. David Perlmutter - A comprehensive guide on the Gut-Brain Connection and how it impacts overall health.

The Mind-Gut Connection: How the Hidden Conversation Within Our Bodies Impacts

Our Mood, Our Choices, and Our Overall Health by Dr. Emeran Mayer - Offers insights into the intricate relationship between the gut and the brain.

The Good Gut: Taking Control of Your Weight, Your Mood, and Your Long-term Health by Justin Sonnenburg and Erica Sonnenburg - Explores the role of the gut microbiome in health and provides actionable advice.

Eat to Beat Disease: The New Science of How Your Body Can Heal Itself by Dr. William W. Li - Covers the latest research on the impact of diet on health and disease prevention.

Websites and Blogs

Harvard Health Blog - Gut Health - Harvard Health Publishing provides expert insights on gut health and its connection to overall well-being.

The Gut-Brain Connection - Johns Hopkins Medicine - A resourceful page explaining the Gut-Brain Connection from a medical perspective.

The Microbiome Report - A blog and podcast dedicated to exploring the world of microbiomes and their impact on health.

Precision Nutrition - All About Gut Health - A comprehensive guide to understanding and improving gut health through nutrition and lifestyle.

Gut-Brain Health Apps and Tools

MyFitnessPal: This app helps you track your food intake, exercise, and overall health, making it easier to monitor your dietary choices.

Calm: Incorporate mindfulness and meditation into your daily routine with the Calm app to manage stress and improve your Gut-Brain Connection.

Headspace: Another excellent mindfulness app that offers guided meditation sessions and techniques for reducing stress.

Welltory: This app measures your stress levels, energy, and overall well-being through heart rate variability analysis, offering insights into the impact of stress on your gut and brain.

Additional Research and Studies

The Gut-Brain Axis: The Missing Link in Depression - A research paper exploring the Gut-Brain Connection and its implications for depression.

Dietary Fiber and Gut Microbiota in Health and Disease - A comprehensive review on the role of dietary fiber in gut health and its impact on various health conditions.

The Role of the Gut Microbiome in Alzheimer's Disease - A study examining the connection between gut microbiota and Alzheimer's disease.

<u>Probiotics in the Treatment of Depression: A Systematic Review</u> - An analysis of the potential use of probiotics in managing depressive symptoms.

These resources will serve as valuable companions on your journey to better gut and brain health. Whether you're seeking further knowledge, practical tools, or the latest research findings, they will aid you in making informed decisions and taking proactive steps towards a healthier and more harmonious Gut-Brain Connection.

Conclusion

In concluding our journey through the intricate world of gut and brain health, we've explored a profound connection that shapes our well-being. Here, we summarize key insights, offer encouragement for your personal Gut-Brain Health journey, and emphasize the transformative power of nutrition in nurturing both your gut and brain.

Summarizing Key Insights

Throughout this book, we've uncovered a wealth of insights:

The Gut-Brain Axis is a dynamic communication network that profoundly influences our health, emotions, and cognitive abilities.

Gut health plays a pivotal role in overall well-being, affecting digestion, immune function, and even mental health.

Nutrition is a cornerstone of Gut-Brain Health, as the foods we eat directly impact our gut microbiota, which, in turn, influences our brain function.

Beneficial dietary choices, including fiber-rich foods, prebiotics, probiotics, and antioxidants, can promote a thriving Gut-Brain Connection.

Lifestyle factors such as exercise, sleep, stress management, and mindfulness significantly contribute to the harmonious operation of the Gut-Brain Axis.

Regular check-ups, preventive measures, and awareness of common digestive disorders are crucial for maintaining long-term gut health.

Encouragement for Embarking on a Gut-Brain Health Journey

Embarking on a Gut-Brain Health journey is a commitment to a healthier, happier life.

It's an endeavor rooted in self-care, and it offers profound benefits for your overall well-being. Remember that progress doesn't require perfection. Small, sustainable changes in your diet, lifestyle, and mindset can lead to remarkable improvements in your Gut-Brain Connection.

As you embark on this journey:

Embrace the power of knowledge. Continue to explore, learn, and stay informed about the latest research and insights into Gut-Brain Health.

Cultivate a sense of mindfulness in your daily life. Pay attention to your body's signals and how the foods you eat make you feel.

Prioritize self-care and stress management. These are fundamental elements of a thriving Gut-Brain Connection.

Seek support and guidance from healthcare professionals, dietitians, and supportive communities to ensure you have the resources and encouragement needed for success.

The Power of Nutrition in Transforming Gut and Brain Health

Nutrition is the cornerstone of your Gut-Brain Health journey. It's the fuel that can either revitalize or hinder the intricate network of communication between your gut and brain. With each meal, you have the opportunity to nourish your microbiota and support your mental and physical well-being.

Embrace the power of nutrition by:

Focusing on a balanced and diverse diet that includes a wide range of whole foods, from colorful fruits and vegetables to lean proteins and whole grains.

Incorporating gut-friendly foods such as fiber-rich options, prebiotics, probiotics, and antioxidants.

Being mindful of the impact of your dietary choices on both your gut and brain health.

Your Gut-Brain Connection is a dynamic and adaptable system. By making conscious and nutritious choices, you can optimize this connection to enjoy a higher quality of life, enhanced mood, and improved cognitive function.

In closing, remember that your journey to improve Gut-Brain Health is a lifelong commitment to well-being. It's a journey filled with delicious foods, mindful moments, and an empowered sense of self. May your Gut-Brain Connection be harmonious, vibrant, and a source of enduring health and vitality.